THEORY DEVELOPMENT
IN NURSING

THEORY DEVELOPMENT IN NURSING

MARGARET A. NEWMAN, Ph.D., R.N., F.A.A.N.
Professor-in-Charge
Graduate Program and Research
Department of Nursing
College of Human Development
The Pennsylvania State University
University Park, Pennsylvania

F. A. DAVIS COMPANY • Philadelphia

Copyright © 1979 by F. A. Davis Company
Second printing 1980
Third printing 1981

All rights reserved. This book is protected by copyright. No part of it may be produced, stored in a retrieval system, or transmitted in any form or by any means, electronic, mechanical, photocopying, recording, or otherwise, without written permission from the publisher.

Printed in the United States of America

Library of Congress Cataloging in Publication Data

Newman, Margaret A
    Theory development in nursing.

    Includes bibliographical references and index.
    1. Nursing—Philosophy.   2. Theory (Philosophy)
I. Title.
RT84.5.N48   610.73'01'9   79-12404
ISBN 0-8036-6520-2

FOREWORD

In 1893, Florence Nightingale claimed that a new art and a new science had been created. She was referring to nursing. The characterization of nursing as an art has seldom been questioned, but to this day it can be questioned whether nursing has yet become a science.

Scientific subjects were a part of the curriculum of the Nightingale school, but the subjects were included so that nurses would understand the "why" of what they were required to do; nursing, however, concerned the "how" and "when" of doing something, a learning of accumulated facts, principles, skills, and techniques. Nurses typically had been taught how, what, and when to do something, and sometimes why, but were seldom taught the process of questioning, conceptualizing, testing, and revising, the essential elements of science.

Nursing has grown as a national resource and has evolved from a procedure- or activity-oriented vocation to a goal-directed professional service for health. The aims and responsibilities of professional nursing and a goal of health require a constantly changing and expanding body of knowledge, knowledge that has been tested and verified through research.

Facts, principles, and subject matter amassed from the past and from a focus on disease are inadequate to meet the full challenge of a science of health or the demands of the winds of change which create obsolescence of ideas as well as technologies. Increasingly, the true professionals in nursing demonstrate that nursing requires intellectual as well as humanitarian activity. They become dissatisfied with the scope and quality of the knowledge base for nursing.

Inadequacies, change, a resurgent orientation to, and redefinition of health, and more comprehensive views of man and environment in interaction have led to attempts to clarify or express the nature of nursing, not only as an activity or an occupation, but also as a field of knowledge. Clarification of the nature of nursing is now essential for the effective organization, development, and transmission of knowledge.

Current formulations or models designed to describe the essential nature or focus of nursing are expressions of the need and search for an orienting and organizing focus or perspective for nursing research and nursing education. Some are offered as organizing frameworks for identifying the essential body of knowledge necessary for effective practice and for identifying and rectifying inadequacies in that knowledge base.

Theory development in nursing arose from the need to

FOREWORD

capture or clarify the nature of nursing. It also grew from increasing discontent among nurses who studied theories and theory development in other disciplines. Such nurses came to realize some inadequacies for nursing purposes in the knowledge from other fields. They came to realize that facts in isolation have little meaning. Facts depend upon a contextual relating to be useful for guiding action. Facts depend upon theories to give them meaning. So also do concepts which have meaning only within the conceptual structures or theories in which they are elements. The dynamic, revisionary nature of knowledge is recognized in nursing, and nurses are experiencing the limitations of extant theories for guiding the actions of today's professional practitioners of nursing.

No longer can professional nurses afford to be enthusiastic but naive and unquestioning consumers of theories and research. They must assume responsibility for the development of nursing theories and the science of nursing, the science which must guide the actions of responsible professionals.

This book makes a singular contribution toward the development of the science of nursing through its clear exposition of the process of theory development within a nursing framework. Theory development, with the reciprocal research, is the process essential for a sound and rational base for contemporary nursing practice and for an effective humanitarian service. Theory development in nursing is the process by which nursing becomes a science and a special type of human caring. Art, sensitivity, and a desire to help are important but are inadequate for effective nursing. Systematized knowledge or science is also essential to turn wishes or intentions into productive action. Humanitarian science through theory development in nursing is a major element in producing effective caring.

Rosemary Ellis, Ph.D., R.N.
Professor of Nursing
Case Western Reserve University
Cleveland, Ohio

CONTENTS

1. INTRODUCTION   1
2. CLARIFICATION OF TERMS   5
3. RELATIONSHIP OF CONCEPTUAL MODELS TO THEORY   15
4. ANALYSIS OF THE THEORETICAL BASIS FOR HYPOTHESIS FORMULATION   23
5. THE PROCESS OF SYNTHESIZING A THEORY   43
6. TOWARD A THEORY OF HEALTH   55
7. SEARCHING FOR MORE HOLISTIC METHODS OF INQUIRY   69

REFERENCES   75
APPENDICES   79
INDEX   87

1
INTRODUCTION

In search of the knowledge which provides the scientific base for nursing, there is a central question: What is nursing theory? Attempts to answer this question raise the underlying questions: What is nursing? What is theory? Although definitions of nursing abound in the literature, they relate primarily to the function of nurses rather than to the content of nursing as a discipline. Consequently, there has been little agreement within the profession as to what constitutes the nature of nursing, a factor which has inhibited progress toward the development of the science of nursing.

Frustrated with attempts to answer the question of what is nursing, attention was switched in more recent years to the question of what is theory. During the past decade explorations have begun regarding the nature of theory and the process of theory development. The contributions of philosophers of science and theorists from other disciplines have been examined in the quest for an understanding of theory, but the utilization of their insights has been incomplete without an adequate conceptualization of nursing.

The answer to the question of what constitutes nursing knowledge was heralded by Florence Nightingale[1] early in the history of the profession, when she pointed out that "The same laws of health, or of nursing, for they are in reality the same, obtain among the well as among the sick." Current nursing theorists agree that the purpose of nursing is the promotion of *health* and that the focus of nursing science is the phenomenon of man. Definitions of health and conceptualizations of man differ in varying degrees and thereby provide the basis for differing theories within the total context of nursing science.

In order for a theory to have direct application to nursing, it must meet the following criteria:

1. The focus is on the life process of man.
2. The purpose is understanding of the patterns of the life process which relate to health.
3. A total elaboration of the theory contains an action component which facilitates health.

These criteria are consistent with the current conceptual models of nursing and include prescriptive level theory, which Dickoff and James[2] consider a necessary component of theory for a profession.

Nursing theories are at various stages of development. Within some conceptual models where the theory is at an early stage of development, activity may be focused on the factor-identification and descriptive levels. In other models, however, the theory is sufficiently developed that

INTRODUCTION

work may proceed at the prescriptive level. Certainly the process does not proceed in a linear fashion but necessitates feedback from all levels in a continuous evaluation of the factors of study and their relationship to health.

The purpose of this book is to try to bring together in a workable whole the various aspects of theory development in nursing: the conceptualizations of nursing which provide the framework for the development of theory, the process one utilizes in specifying a testable theory, and some suggested methods which are particularly applicable to research in nursing.

In the following chapter, the terms which will be used are defined. The details regarding propositional statements may not have relevance for the reader who is confronting this material for the first time, but an understanding of these details is necessary when the actual process of theory construction is taking place. Although this aspect of the process logically follows, rather than precedes, an understanding of the conceptual framework within which one is working, it seemed necessary to present this material first. Some readers may prefer to skip to Chapter 3 on conceptual models and then return to Chapter 2.

In Chapter 3, selected conceptual models are examined as to the direction they provide for nursing theory development. It is not the intent of this book to address all of the nursing models which have been developed, but rather to illustrate the differences in some of the current models and how they relate to the direction and stage of theory development within the model. Presented here is a comparison of the essential components of the models elaborated by Dorothy Johnson, Martha Rogers, and Sister Callista Roy. Both Johnson and Rogers have been pioneers in providing a foundation for the development of nursing theory; Roy's model, a more recent contribution to the field, has been widely utilized as a basis for practice and curriculum development.

Chapter 4 contains an analysis of the process of theory construction as a basis for the formulation of hypotheses. The studies chosen as a basis for analysis illustrate the logic of this process and, at the same time, pose some of the problems often encountered.

In Chapter 5, there is an attempt to share with the reader the steps one goes through in undertaking the process of developing a theory. If this chapter is not clear and complete, one reason is that the process is not always clear and the product is never complete. Another is a reflection of my own stage of development as nursing theorist.

In order for the conceptualization of nursing to be complete and to provide a framework for the development of theory, there must be an adequate conceptualization of health. Chapter 6 presents my view of health and outlines a set of interrelated propositions which can provide the basis for testing and further elaboration.

The final chapter represents an initial exploration of the task confronting nursing scientists: to develop not only the directions of nursing's inquiry, but also methods appropriate to the discipline.

2

CLARIFICATION OF TERMS

There is a great deal of ambiguity in the use of terms such as theory, conceptual framework, theoretical framework, and so on. When clarification of what is meant by these terms is required, it is often apparent that they are being used interchangeably and are sufficiently vague as to have little meaning.

The term conceptual framework seems to be particularly vulnerable to different interpretations. Some people will refer to a conceptual framework which has been elaborated by a particular theorist as "Dr. X's *theory*." Even Dr. X may refer to the conceptual framework alternately as a conceptual system, conceptual model, or theoretical system or framework. In addition, one will often find a section in the report of research entitled "Conceptual Framework," which seems to denote the broad, general theoretical context that provides the background for the study.

From my standpoint, the terms conceptual framework and conceptual model may be used interchangeably and represent a matrix of concepts which together describe the focus of inquiry. Hempel[3] specifies that these concepts are linked together by broad generalizations; however, these linkages may or may not be explicit in the initial elaboration of the system. A conceptual framework may be visualized as an umbrella with its hub representing the focus of inquiry and the outer points representing the major concepts. The lines connecting the points to the hub and to each other would represent the broad generalizations.

The purpose of a conceptual framework is to provide a focus which directs the questions one asks and the theories one proposes and subsequently tests. It provides a network within which questions, theories, and data fit together and makes possible the identification of needed areas of theory development. Such a system cannot be regarded as a theory because it, in itself, does not provide an explanation of the phenomenon in question and is not testable. Since it is not testable, its viability rests primarily in its usefulness in generating relevant theory. If the assumptions of the system become untenable or the level of generalization is insufficient, the conceptual framework may fall into disuse.

A theory, in contrast, is testable and, therefore, refutable and alterable. Popper[4] states that a theory may be "one powerful, unifying idea," and as such the term theory can apply to an explanation of the relationship between only two concepts, e.g., the relativity of space and time. As a theory develops, however, it contains more specific information, and a series of interrelated propositions emerge. From such a set of propositions, which may be considered a theoretical framework or system, new relationships may be deduced and tested, and the data therefrom then will

CLARIFICATION OF TERMS

either strengthen or weaken the theoretical system from which the tested relationship is drawn. The process is continuous and, therefore, the nature of the knowledge is always changing, at some times more rapidly than at others.

The fluid nature of the body of knowledge called nursing science is often difficult to accept. For those who have been indoctrinated with hard and fast rules, or at least the idea that a body of knowledge is solid, it is not easy to become comfortable with the idea that science is a process more often concerned with asking questions than with finding answers. Science is the process of knowing, the process of finding out about a particular phenomenon, and in the case of nursing science, it is the process of finding out how to facilitate the health of man. Theory utilized in practice must of necessity be subjected to repeated tests and must stand the test of time. From that standpoint, the changing nature of nursing theory may not be apparent. In the initial stages of the development of a theory, however, the theory may be overthrown immediately. Even if the relationship posed by the theory does not hold up under testing, this finding contributes to an explanation of the phenomenon and is an important part of the process.

Since a theory states a specific relationship between two or more concepts, definitions of a concept and related terms are necessary.

A *concept* is an abstraction formed by generalization from particulars. For example, consider the concept of a table. Each person has an idea of what represents a table. It could be defined as a piece of furniture with a horizontal plane for the purpose of supporting other objects. To go further than that and be specific about what kind of table one has in mind would alter the concept in terms of observable characteristics, such as the number of legs the table has, the shape of the table, and so on. If these specific characteristics were added to the original definition of the concept of table, a *construct* would be formed. A construct incorporates the meaning of the concept but modifies it by limiting the concept to certain observable characteristics by which the concept may be measured, thereby making it amenable to testing. The measurement of the construct often results in a symbolic range of numbers, such as in the case of the above example, the area of the table. At this point, one is dealing with a *variable*. In research, the term "variable" is used to refer to both the major concepts of the study and also the intervening concepts; however, in the strictest sense of the term, it refers to the numbers representing the concepts. One can readily see from this example that there can be many constructs of the same concept and that studies based on different constructs may not be testing the same phenomenon, even though the concept may be defined similarly. Moreover, the concept itself may be defined differently, but in the modification of the concept for testing purposes, the variables being tested are the same, e.g., different concepts of anxiety tested by the same test of anxiety. The greater the discrepancy between the concept and the construct, the less one is testing the main theory, i.e., the relationship of the concepts. Since the main theory describes the relationship in abstract terms, it is not testable; therefore, one must resort to the testing of an auxiliary theory composed of constructs. The resulting data will be

CLARIFICATION OF TERMS 9

in terms of variables which are amenable to statistical analysis.

Theories are stated in the form of *propositions*. A proposition is a specific relationship between two or more concepts. This definition may be confusing, since it has already been used to describe a theory. The difference is that a theory *may* consist of only one proposition but more often is composed of a set of interrelated propositions.

Dubin[5] distinguishes between what he calls a law of interrelationship and a proposition. The former is more general and specifies what the relationship is; the latter includes specific values and states the predicted values of the units. The following is a law of interrelationship:

> Anxiety is positively related to a personal (1)
> space preference.

Whereas a proposition based on that relationship might be:

> As level of anxiety increases, there will be (2)
> a preference for increased personal space.

Blalock[6] emphasizes the necessity of specifying the direction of the relationship, i.e., whether it is symmetrical or asymmetrical. The above proposition (2) implies an asymmetrical relationship, i.e., the direction of the relationship is one-way; it proceeds from a change in anxiety level to a change in preference for personal space, and not the other way around. The law of interrelationship (1), however, does not specify the direction of the relationship and could be interpreted to be symmetrical, meaning that a change in either of the concepts will have a direct relationship on the other. If this reciprocal type of relationship is not the intent of the writer, it should be made clear in the statement of the relationship. The law of interrelationship (1) could be restated as follows:

A change in anxiety will produce a direct change in preference for personal space.

Propositions, in order to satisfy this criterion on directionality, may be stated as follows:

If there is a change in $\vec{A}$, then there will be a change in B.

or

A change in $\vec{A}$ leads to (produces) a change in B.

or

A change in $\overset{\leftarrow}{B}$ is a function of a change in A.

Each of the above statements indicates a specific direction (illustrated by arrows) for the relationship, which is asymmetrical. In addition, as much as possible, the value of the concepts (represented by the letters A and B) should be specified, and further, if possible, the boundaries of these values. For instance, in curvilinear relationships, the values of the two terms change at a certain point: an increase in anxiety may lead to an increase in learning *up to a point*

CLARIFICATION OF TERMS 11

at which further increase in anxiety may lead to a decrement in learning.

The terminology used in specifying the direction of relationship within the proposition implies causality, and that is not what is intended. I know of no other way, at the present time, of attaining the precision we are seeking in theory development than to specify that a relationship flows one way and not the other, if that is what the evidence from the literature indicates. Otherwise, we will find ourselves pursuing even more dead ends than we do under the best of circumstances.

The following diagrams, utilizing letters to present the units, or concepts, of a theory, will illustrate how different interpretations of the direction of the relationships posed by the propositions will result in different derivations of relationships to be tested. If the reality* of a situation were:

1. An increase in A leads to an increase in B.
 ($\uparrow A \rightarrow \uparrow B$)
2. An increase in B leads to an increase in C.
 ($\uparrow B \rightarrow \uparrow C$)
3. An increase in C leads to an increase in D.
 ($\uparrow C \rightarrow \uparrow D$)

These propositions could then be diagrammed:

$$\uparrow A \rightarrow \uparrow B \rightarrow \uparrow C \rightarrow \uparrow D$$

---

*This example is, of course, an oversimplification of reality, since reality, if it were known, would contain multiple variables interacting in ways unknown to the observer. This example is used simply to illustrate the necessity of directionality in propositions.

from which one could derive the following new relationships:

4. An increase in A leads to an increase in C.
5. An increase in A leads to an increase in D.   (Set I)
6. An increase in B leads to an increase in D.

If the author of the original propositions had been vague and failed to specify the direction of the relationships, someone else might have interpreted them to be symmetrical, or reciprocal, relationships, and a diagram of such relationships

$$\uparrow A \leftrightarrows \uparrow B \leftrightarrows \uparrow C \leftrightarrows \uparrow D$$

would result in different derivations. In addition to the three relationships derived from the asymmetrical set of propositions, the following relationships may be derived from the symmetrical set:

7. An increase in C leads to an increase in A.
8. An increase in D leads to an increase in A.   (Set II)
9. An increase in D leads to an increase in B.

Since the testing of the relationship between two concepts establishes *only* the presence or absence of a *relationship* and not the direction of the relationship, a correlational test of the relationships, specified in Sets I and II, would produce the same results. However, if the erroneous direction of the derived relationships in Set II is maintained in subsequent sets of propositions from which new relationships are derived, it may lead to faulty derivations, and the error compounds itself.

CLARIFICATION OF TERMS 13

Two other terms, *axiom* and *theorem*, have been used by Blalock to distinguish between the propositions one chooses as the basis for one's theory and the propositions which are derived from this theoretical framework. The propositions which form the set of interrelated relationships are specific in terms of the direction of the relationships and are *assumed** to be true; they are referred to as the axioms of the theory. The propositions which can be derived from this set of axioms are converted into statements of relationship, without causal implication, for the purpose of testing the relationship. These derived testable relationships are referred to as theorems.

In summary, a conceptual model (framework) specifies the focus of inquiry for the discipline. Within the framework, major concepts are identified and basic assumptions about the phenomenon of inquiry are explicated. The major concepts and basic assumptions provide direction for the identification of subconcepts and the specification of theories relating these concepts to each other. As sets of related concepts emerge, new relationships may be derived. Partial testing of theories is possible by the utilization of constructs, which modify the concepts in measurable terms.

---

*This assumption is very different from a basic assumption, which refers to a statement accepted as true on the basis of abundant evidence of those universal-type truths. The assumption of truth made in the choice of axioms is simply for the purpose of linking together propositions from which new relationships may be derived. The statements may or may not in actuality be "true."

3

RELATIONSHIP OF CONCEPTUAL MODELS TO THEORY

Conceptual models provide a way of looking at things. As already stated, a conceptual model is not a theory in the strictest sense of the term but constitutes a framework which focuses our thinking in a particular way.

In a practice discipline, conceptual models are useful both in directing the work of scientists in the development of theories and in directing the observations of practitioners as the process of assessment and intervention is carried out. As various conceptual models have been proposed for nursing, differences become apparent in terms of the focus (the phenomenon under scrutiny), the underlying assumptions, definitions of health and illness, and designation of the goal of nursing. It is important to examine the differences and consider what ramifications they may have in the development of nursing knowledge.

COMPARISON OF BASIC COMPONENTS OF SELECTED MODELS

As one examines the basic components of the models of Johnson,[7] Roy,[8] and Rogers[9] (see Appendix A), it can be seen that all three theorists focus on man in constant interaction with the environment, but the way in which they have conceptualized man and the nature of that interaction differs. Johnson describes man as a "behavioral system composed of interrelated parts" (or subsystems) which form "an organized and integrated whole."[7,10] She depicts the whole by designation of the parts. Roy, too, by virtue of the way in which she expresses her view of man, i.e., a biopsychosocial being, proceeds in the same direction and depicts man as a integration of biological and social components. Rogers, on the other hand, begins with the whole and specifies that this approach describes a phenomenon that possesses characteristics which are more than and different from the sum of the parts.

While Johnson sees the behavior of man as being patterned and repetitive and striving toward behavioral system balance as an adaptation to impinging environmental forces, Rogers asserts that what appears to be repetition is only similarity and that the life process of the individual is manifesting itself in emerging *new* patterns which are moving toward increasing complexity, not toward equilibrium and stability. Although Johnson sees behavioral system equilibrium as essential to man, she goes on to say that man seeks new experiences which may disturb his steady state temporarily, and she sees nursing as promoting *dynamic* stability. The dynamic quality which she as-

CONCEPTUAL MODELS AND THEORY

signs to equilibrium and the seeking of new experiences may be congruent with Rogers' idea of increasing complexity. Nevertheless, both Johnson and Roy assert that man must adapt, and must adapt "successfully" or positively, to environmental changes, whereas Rogers is consistent in her assumption that the changes taking place in man are a manifestation of mutual, simultaneous interaction between man and his environment, with the implication that no value is assigned to the nature of the interaction. Later, however, Rogers does differentiate patterns of interaction as enhancing or disruptive of man's development.

In describing the nature of the interaction process, Johnson emphasizes the characteristics of man, i.e., the behavioral responses developed through maturation and experience and governed by biological, psychological, and social factors. Roy utilizes Helson's model of adaptation as a function of focal, contextual, and residual stimuli. Roy's approach takes into consideration the characteristics of both the individual and the environment and on the surface might appear similar to Rogers' approach, that is, that change depends on the state of the human field and the simultaneous state of the environmental field; however, the emphasis in Roy's approach on the focal stimulus has the tendency of focusing thinking on the most prominent stimulus, and hence reaction to it, rather than a total view, as advocated by Rogers.

The ways in which these theorists view the man-environment interaction, together with their concepts of health and illness, influence the focus which they specify for nursing. Johnson defines nursing as:

... an external regulatory force which acts to preserve the organization and integration of the patient's behavior under those conditions *in which illness is found.* [emphasis mine]

Roy states that nursing:

... focuses on the patient as a person adapting to those stimuli present as a result of his position on the health-illness continuum.

The health-illness continuum, in Roy's view, ranges from very healthy to very ill. Rogers, on the other hand, views health and illness as:

... expressions of the process of life. Their meaning is derived out of an understanding of the life process in its totality.

Consistent with this view, Rogers then states that nursing:

... focuses on human beings—on man in his entirety and wholeness.

... encompasses the man-environmental relationship and seeks to identify sequential, cross-sectional patterning in the life process.

It can be seen from these definitions that the Johnson and Roy models describe nursing as assisting individuals in their response to illness, whereas the Rogers model depicts nursing as identifying patterns of the life process. All three models depict nursing as seeking to promote a more

CONCEPTUAL MODELS AND THEORY 19

effective way of life for the individual. Johnson specifies nursing's contribution to patient welfare as:

> ... that of fostering efficient and effective behavioral functioning in the patient to prevent illness and during and following illness.

Roy specifies that the goal of nursing is:

> ... to bring about an adapted state in the patient which frees him to respond to other stimuli present.

Rogers asserts that nursing:

> ... is directed toward repatterning of man and environment for more effective fulfillment of life's capabilities.

> ... seeks to promote symphonic interaction between man and environment, to strengthen the coherence and integrity of the human field, and to direct and redirect patterning of the human and environmental fields for realization of maximum health potential.

The goals, therefore, of the models appear to be very similar. The basic beliefs about health and illness, however, differ and result in different ways of viewing the phenomena in question. The Johnson and Roy models present a problem-oriented approach, and each of these theorists provides a framework for assessing the state of the individual. Roy identifies her model as a practice model, and knowledge basic to assessment within her framework derives from the biological, psychological, and social sciences. Johnson's model incorporates more specific categories of assessment, but she agrees that the basic factors are biological, psychological, and social.

Although Rogers sees the theory which derives from her conceptual model as capable of being translated into practice, she is the least clear regarding a framework for assessment. This vagueness may be related to the fact that the primary purpose of her model, as she sees it, is for the generation of knowledge incorporating a totally different view of man. She has specified what the basic assumptions are in relation to this view—holism, open systems, increasing complexity, unidirectionality, pattern and organization—but she is not specific regarding the major concepts which describe the life process.

DIRECTIONS FOR THEORY DEVELOPMENT

Both the Johnson and Roy models utilize a framework based on knowledge developed in other disciplines. The language of these models is familiar, and, therefore, they are readily adaptable as a guide for practice and curriculum development.

Theory development within the framework of these models falls primarily into two categories. The first is an extension of the current theory from the psychological, sociological, and biological sciences as they relate to the assessment categories of the models. This type of theory would be at the predictive level. The second would be a testing of the action component of these models to determine whether or not the criterion for successful, or positive, adaptation has been accomplished. In Johnson's model, the author implies that when the goals of the system (meaning man as a behavioral system) are met, the outcome will be economy of energy, efficiency of action, and facilitation of social interaction. Roy asserts that actions which bring about an adapted state will release energy for the healing process and enable the individual to respond to an increased number of stimuli. Whether or not these goals are indeed accomplished by particular nursing actions requires systematic testing. This type of theory would be at the prescriptive level.

Rogers' conceptual model calls for a completely different way of viewing man and his world. Since her framework represents a revolution of a sort, theory development within her framework is in a rudimentary stage, and, therefore, must proceed at the beginning levels of Dickoff and James' categorization before proceeding to the prescriptive level. Since Rogers has not specified what she considers to be the major concepts of her system, that task is still to be accomplished. The question to be asked in attempting to identify a concept for exploration is: Does it satisfy the basic assumptions of the model? For instance, can it be considered a manifestation of wholeness? Does it reflect a pattern and organization which is specific to the individual? Do the pattern and organization reflect rhythmicity and unidirectionality?

In calling for a new way of viewing man, as well as health and illness, Rogers' model does not require that one discard previous knowledge, but it does require that such knowledge be viewed differently. Disease conditions can no longer be considered as entities unto themselves but must be regarded as manifestations of the total pattern of the individual in interaction with the environment. The knowledge that is sought is an understanding of the man-environment patterns of energy exchange.

4

ANALYSIS OF THE THEORETICAL BASIS FOR HYPOTHESIS FORMULATION

In order for nursing research to have meaning in terms of theory development, it must (1) have as its purpose the testing of theory, (2) make explicit the theoretical framework upon which the testing relies, and (3) re-examine the theoretical underpinnings in light of the findings. In addition, and of great importance, the process of theory development requires many studies examining as many relationships as possible regarding a particular concept. In order for progress to take place within a reasonable period of time, it is essential that investigators systematically consider the interrelationships of their findings and the meaning they have in the formulation of a theory.

Analysis of another investigator's work can be helpful in identifying the necessary ingredients in the process of theory development and testing. Two of the questions to be asked are:

What propositions can be drawn from the author's review of the literature?

What is the strength of the evidence for such propositions?

Often, in the translation of the author's work into propositions, it is necessary to draw one's own conclusions about the meaning and direction of the relationship, and it may be impossible at that point to evaluate the strength of the relationship. Blalock[6] advises:

> As the process of diagramming a particular author's argument is taking place, there will undoubtedly be a number of ambiguities that will arise, some of which may not have been previously noted. Did the author intend that the implied relationship is direct or mediated through some other variable in the system? Is the direction of causality implied? Is there any indication that the predicted relationship is nonlinear? Does the effect take place quickly, or with a lengthy delay? Are other variables introduced as qualifying variables, and if so, are these explicitly linked to any other variables in the system?
>
> In asking such questions, one must allow for the possibility that an author's discussion is too vague or ambiguous to permit a definite answer. At this point, one may be tempted to make a thorough search of the author's work to obtain an answer. Such a search may very well prove fruitless, or it may be found that the author has been inconsistent or deliberately ambiguous. At the risk of being accused of professional heresy, I would suggest that in such instances one should forget what the theorist intended—even though he be a very renowned scholar—and that one insert his own theoretical linkages. Otherwise, he may become prematurely immersed in 'scholarship,' in the worst sense of the term. [p. 29]

BASIS FOR HYPOTHESIS FORMULATION

An analysis of the theoretical framework of Schlachter's[11] investigation of anxiety and personal space provides the basis for evaluating the relationship of the process of theory construction to the formulation of hypotheses. In Table 1, selected statements from the review of literature in Schlachter's study have been translated into propositions. The reader will note that I have taken the liberty of categorizing and renaming some of the concepts and have made explicit the direction of the relationships. No attempt has been made to evaluate the strength or the "truth" of the asserted relationships. At this point they are taken at face value as part of the author's argument; later, in the evaluation of the findings and in the subsequent development of the theory, one would find it necessary to attend to this crucial aspect of the process.

The 26 propositions which can be derived from the literature make the task of evaluating the theoretical framework a more manageable one, but further consolidation is needed. Now the questions to be asked are:

Are there propositions which are similar enough in meaning that can be combined into one?

Are there any apparent linkages between propositions?

At this point, it may be helpful to begin to develop diagrams of the relationships depicted in the propositions. Schlachter specified four major constructs: anxiety, perceived personal space, perceived body space, and actual body space (see Appendix B). The relational statements included in her literature review were grouped according

TABLE 1. Propositions Based on Literature Review in Schlachter's Study of Anxiety and Personal Space

Excerpts from Literature Review*	Derived Propositions
Physiologically it [anxiety] if manifested by increased adrenocortical function, increased muscle tension, increased heart rate and cardiac output, and palmar sweat determinations.	1. Anxiety produces sympathoadrenal-medullary response.
... stress situations induce anxiety. ...	2. Environmental stress produces anxiety.
... simple withdrawal is a fundamental type of reaction of stress ... in addition to withdrawing physically, the individual may withdraw in various psychological ways. ...	3. Stress leads to physical and psychological withdrawal.
May describes various forms of avoidance in the presence of anxiety, and notes that the behavior is manifested in flight, helplessness, or flight patterns.	4. Anxiety produces avoidance behavior.
Subjects report external symptoms such as neurodermatitis and rheumatoid arthritis when the body is viewed as a barrier in the presence of anxiety. Other subjects who have a concept of the body as permeable report the involvement of visceral organs in the presence of anxiety. ...	5. If the body is viewed as a barrier, anxiety produces external physiological changes. 6. If the body is viewed as permeable, anxiety produces internal physiological changes.
... with anxiety, the individual becomes more alert and experiences heightened self-awareness, but that at the same time the perceptual field is often narrowed; however, as the anxiety increases, the subject is less able to differentiate between himself and objects.	7. Moderate levels of anxiety produce increased alertness and self-awareness combined with narrowed perceptual field.

BASIS FOR HYPOTHESIS FORMULATION

TABLE 1. *Continued.*

Excerpts from Literature Review	*Derived Propositions*
	8. High levels of anxiety produce decreased differentiation of self from environment.
... if the individual is subjected to stress and anxiety is produced ... his spatial and temporal concepts will be modified as a result of the introduction of anxiety.	9. Anxiety as a result of environmental stress will produce changes in spatial and temporal perception.
... the [body] position maintained by the subject is related to whether or not the subject is anxious.	10. Anxiety affects body position.
... if anxiety, as defined by a lack of mutual trust, is present ... loss of eye contact, backing away from the investigator, and repositioning of the subjects are noted.	11. Anxiety produces avoidance behavior.
... under stressful conditions the dolphins tend to spend more time in tight schools; under nonstressful conditions the social distance is increased.	12. In dolphins, environmental stress produces decreased social distance.
... a decrease in distance and noticeable relaxation of the body angle are significant indexes of liking for the addressee.	13. If there is liking for addressee, decreased social distance will be maintained.
... neurologic lesions of the parietal lobes of the brain often lead to changes in the individual's conceptualization of his body.	14. Neurological changes in the brain lead to changes in body concept.
... body distortion increases with the occurrence of lesions in the supramarginal gyri of the brain.	

TABLE 1. *Continued.*

Excerpts from Literature Review	Derived Propositions
... the individaul's psychological and physiological states are involved in the perception and the possible distortion of perception of his body.	15. Psychological and physiological states affect body concept.
... the body is the meeting ground of physiology and psychology; therefore, a distortion in either will result in a distortion of corporeal awareness.	16. Psychological or physiological distortion produces distortion of body concept.
... body image or any component part of it may change from one situation to another.	17. Situational changes may lead to changes in body image.
... subjects with low-barrier [body boundary] scores were more susceptible to heart rate changes [via conditioning] than those subjects with high-barrier scores.	18. If there is diminished definiteness of body boundary, an individual is more susceptible to imposed alterations in autonomic functioning.
... psychologic distortion such as that present in schizophrenia was related to body-image distortion in that these patients often lost cognizance of body boundaries to the extent that they reported room boundaries as their own.	19. Psychological distortion leads to diminished awareness of body boundaries (extension of self to environmental boundaries).
... the body boundaries perceived by individuals are part of the acquired body image....	20. Body boundaries are a component of body image.
... the immediate physical proximity of another object had a definite effect on the individual's concept of body size.	21. Distance from another object effects body concept in terms of size.

BASIS FOR HYPOTHESIS FORMULATION

TABLE 1. *Continued.*

Excerpts from Literature Review	*Derived Propositions*
... the definiteness of body boundaries appears to be closely related to the ability of the subjects to visualize themselves as individuals.	22. Ability to visualize self as an individual (level of self-differentiation) affects definiteness of body boundaries.
... perception of body size varied with the degree of obesity.	23. Obesity affects body concept in terms of size.
... variations in personal space concepts present in diverse cultures.	24. Personal space concepts are a function of culture.
... when perception is disturbed and the individual views himself as contiguous with the field, personal space might well incorporate the field. On the other hand, when one is able to perceive himself as separate and distinct from the environment, perceived personal space may be diminished.	25. Increased differentiation of self from environment leads to decreased perceived personal space. *or* Level of self-differentiation has an indirect effect on perceived personal space.
... violent individuals are much more sensitive to physical closeness than non-violent individuals.	26. Violent tendencies produce need for increased personal space.

*Schlachter, L.: *The Relation Between Anxiety, Perceived Body and Personal Space and Actual Body Space Among Young Female Adults.* Ph.D. dissertation, New York University, 1971.

to the first three of these constructs; therefore, the initial diagrams might look like those depicted in Figure 1. Apparently, Schlachter is utilizing literature regarding body concept (image) as a background for her construct, perceived body space, and in the statement of her hypotheses (see Appendix B), she seems to be attempting to measure the concept of distortion of body image by combining perceived body space with actual body space. Nevertheless, from the propositions given in Figure 1, one can now begin to link together the major concepts of the study.

There are two pathways through which anxiety may relate to body image: by the physiological changes taking place or by the psychological ones, more specifically the changes in ability to differentiate self. Only one clear pathway between anxiety and personal space is apparent, through self-differentiation; however, a couple of others lend support to a direct relationship between the two, i.e., avoidance behavior and Proposition 13, in which the implicit assumption is that nonliking for addressee is stress-provoking. It is now possible to eliminate, for the time being, propositions which do not appear to be crucial to the theoretical framework (but which will be important in the research design) and summarize the set of propositions which appear to make up the foundation of new and testable theorems:

1. Environmental stress produces an increase in anxiety.
2. Increased anxiety produces a physiological response known as sympathoadrenal-medullary response.

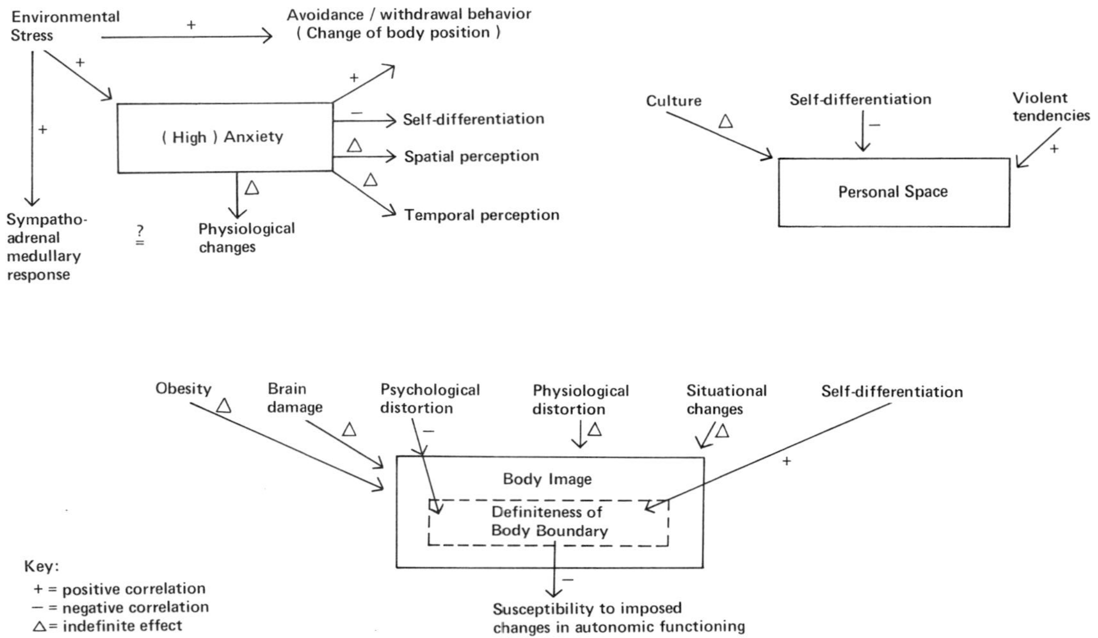

FIGURE 1. Diagram of propositions based on Schlachter's literature review (1971).

3. High levels of anxiety produce decreased self-differentiation.
4. Physiological changes produce a change in body image.
5. Self-differentiation has a direct effect on definiteness of body boundaries.
6. Self-differentiation has a negative effect on perceived personal space.

A diagram of these propositions, which now can be regarded as axioms, appears in Figure 2. Utilizing the pathways charted in this diagram, one can see that it is possible to derive several new relationships:

1. Environmental stress is related negatively to definiteness of body boundaries.
2. Environmental stress is related negatively to self-differentiation.
3. Environmental stress is related positively to perceived personal space.
4. High anxiety is related to decreased definiteness of body boundaries.
5. High anxiety is related positively to perceived personal space.

Since Schlachter chose to focus on anxiety as the independent variable in her study, the relationships posited in 4 and 5 above are the ones which the analysis would indicate are derivable from the theoretical background. The main theory is that a high level of anxiety will bring about a decrease in the definiteness of body boundaries and an increase in the personal space zone an individual

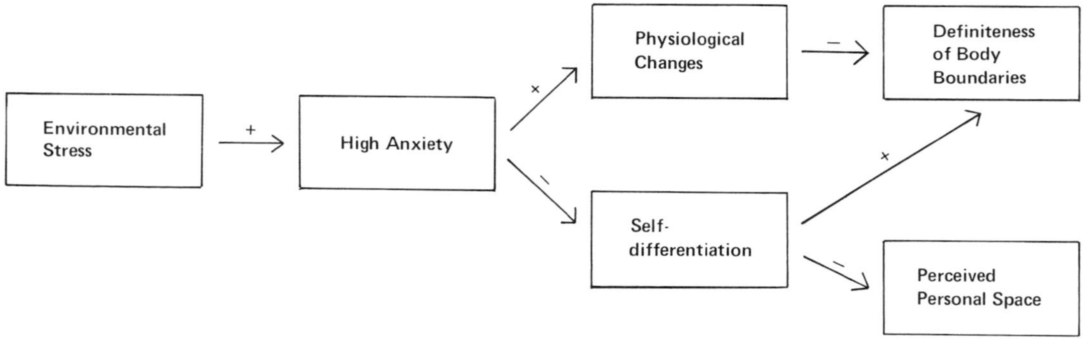

FIGURE 2. Diagram of axioms based on Schlachter's literature review (1971).

maintains and that these changes are mediated through the physiological changes occurring in conjunction with high anxiety states and/or through decreased differentiation of self. The auxiliary theory, composed of constructs, makes testing possible (see Fig. 3).

In the main theory, physiological response and self-differentiation are included as intervening variables, and since intervening variables may or may not be tested, they are omitted in the auxiliary theory, and in their place there is an indication that there may be other intervening variables that the author has not identified. Moreover, in the auxiliary theory, other arrows are included to illustrate that there may be many other variables which are essential to the theory but which as yet have not been identified. An example of this latter point can be seen in the diagram of axioms drawn from the author's literature review. It may be possible that the high level of anxiety needed in order to bring about the physiological and psychological changes through which body boundaries and personal space are affected does not occur unless in combination with an environmental stressor. If this is so and the environmental stress is not present in the testing situation, then the relationship between anxiety and the other variables may not be supported.

Another factor which must be taken into consideration when evaluating the extent to which the theory is being tested is the distance that is imposed between the main theory and the auxiliary theory by the method of measurement. The measurement device reduces the concept to something tangible and may grasp only a small portion of the true nature of the concept. Therefore the testing of the auxiliary theory cannot be regarded as a true test of

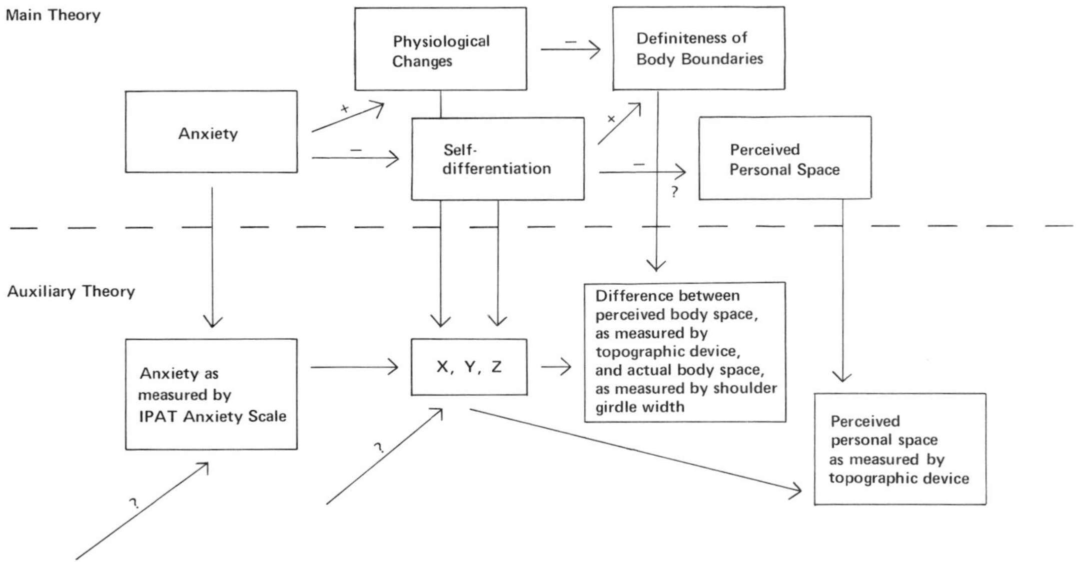

Main Theory

Auxiliary Theory

FIGURE 3. Illustration of proposed main theory and auxiliary theory in Schlachter's study of personal space.

the main theory, and one must be content with partial testing and partial "truth."

The reader will undoubtedly have some objections to the relationships posited by the literature review or think of others which should have been included. At the same time, one may disagree with the way in which propositions were consolidated or the pathways which were chosen as linkages of the theory. These differences of opinion or viewpoint really do not matter for the purpose of understanding the process and utilizing it to evaluate the work of others. On the contrary, being able to identify the weak links, omissions, or false directions in the interrelationships which comprise the theory is the purpose of the endeavor and makes possible the revision and strengthening of the theory each time it is scrutinized.

In Schlachter's work, it is difficult to continue with the third aspect of the analysis, i.e., re-examination of the theory in light of the findings, since she chose to group the dependent variables in combination with each other and did not test directly the relationships posed in Figure 3. Another study of personal space, by Rodgers,[12] provides the basis for this aspect of the analysis. Again, the propositions based on the literature and stated as axioms may or may not have been the intent of the author, but represent my interpretation of her theoretical framework. The following propositions may be drawn from her literature review and appear to be the axioms:

1. If there is a high level of sociability, there is decreased personal space.
2. If there is a high level of sociability, there is an increased arousal threshold.

BASIS FOR HYPOTHESIS FORMULATION

3. An increased arousal threshold is associated with a decreased arousal level.
4. Arousal level has a direct effect on efficiency.
5. Arousal level is a function of time of day.

Figure 4 presents these propositions schematically.

Rodgers hypothesizes that all subjects will prefer more personal space in the morning as compared to the evening and that persons low in sociability will prefer more personal space than persons high in sociability. Both of these relationships appear, from the author's argument, to be mediated through level of arousal; however, the linkage between level of arousal and personal space is only implied, and there is some evidence that sociability is linked directly to personal space. Assuming that Rodgers did intend to include level of arousal as the pathway through which sociability and time of day influence personal space, a diagram of her theory is illustrated in Figure 5.

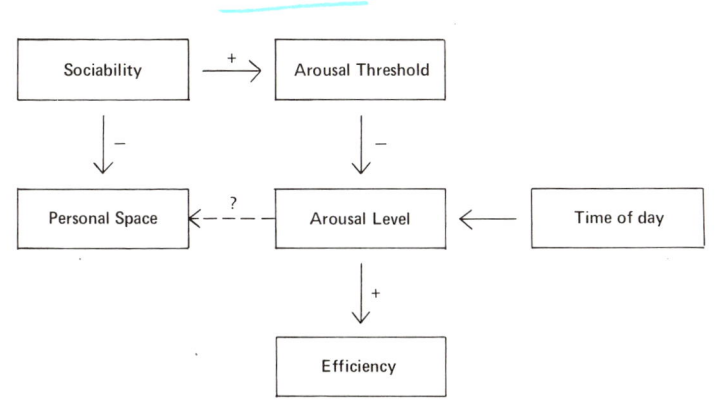

FIGURE 4. Diagram of axioms based on Rodgers' literature review (1971).

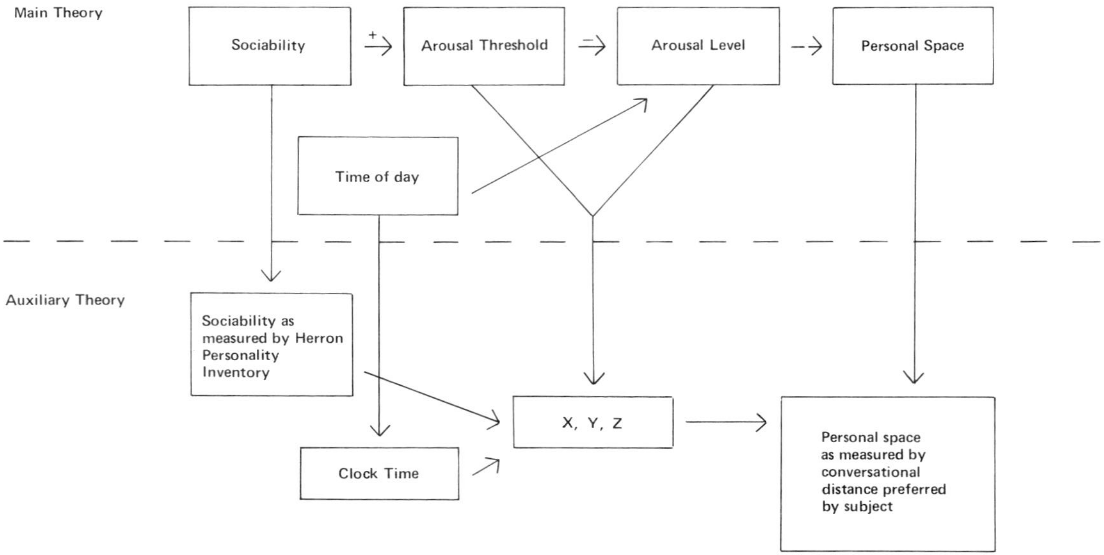

FIGURE 5. Illustration of proposed main theory and auxiliary theory in Rodgers' study of personal space.

BASIS FOR HYPOTHESIS FORMULATION 39

Rodgers' hypotheses tested, among other things, the relationship between (1) sociability and personal space and between (2) time of day and personal space. The data supported the latter hypothesis but not the former. She did not choose to measure level of arousal, through which the relationship of the major concepts was mediated. Since the level of arousal varies from person to person (some people are more alert in the morning, others at night, and so on), there is no way to know whether or not the data of this study support the theory.

Even though it is not necessary to test the intervening variables of a theory (and, indeed, it is not possible even to identify all of the factors), in this particular case it seems crucial to the interpretation of the data. By testing level of arousal, it would be possible to determine:

1. Whether or not a relationship between level of arousal and personal space exists.
2. Whether or not a relationship between sociability and personal space exists independent of level of arousal or only in connection with level of arousal.
3. Whether or not the relationship between time of day and personal space is a function of level of arousal.

This example illustrates the value of specifying the pathways by which one postulates that certain relationships exist, so that steps may be taken in the design and testing to account for as many alternatives as possible and thereby provide more information about the theory.

Finally, the need for establishing the relatedness of studies based on the same concept has become apparent among nursing researchers. Series of studies are beginning to emerge which build on each other, most often with one principal investigator at the helm, as well as cluster studies conducted by a number of investigators on the same topic at the same time. Also emerging, though less often employed, is the deliberate building of one study upon another by different investigators at different times and places. By this building on, I do not mean simply utilizing the results of another's study as part of the theoretical background of a study. I mean more specifically utilizing the same construct and axioms of a theory and re-examining questionable linkages or adding new concepts to strengthen and build the theory.

Consider again the work of Schlachter and Rodgers. Since these two investigators were conducting their studies concurrently in isolation from each other, it cannot be expected that their constructs would be identical, and they were not, as shown below:

Schlachter	Rodgers
Perceived personal space: that area perceived by the subject as being the space usually maintained between himself and another individual and having its periphery identified by means of a topographic device.	*Personal space:* the amount of distance an individual prefers between himself and another for comfortable conversation (measured as inches between subject and experimenter).

Although the authors appeared to be interested in the same concept, both the meaning and the measurement of their constructs differ, and these differences are merely a

BASIS FOR HYPOTHESIS FORMULATION

beginning when one starts to review the literature on personal space.

In the initial development of theories it may be necessary to overlook some of the differences in constructs and to be satisfied with gross approximations of the nature of relationships. Ideally, however, investigators interested in the same concept could develop a kind of master plan in which the same construct is utilized, with each investigator working on different portions of the theory. As sets of interrelated propositions emerge and are tested, the findings therefrom can be utilized to re-evaluate the proposed linkages of the theoretical system and to identify additional relationships. In this way the data from hypothesis testing provide feedback to the theoretical system, and the system is modified and refined accordingly.

5

THE PROCESS OF SYNTHESIZING A THEORY

In theory development, there is no set place marked "go." Some prefer the inductive method, others the deductive method, and still others a combination of the two. Perhaps process is the key word, and, as has been said about research, the process is rarely orderly. However, one has to begin somewhere, and a good place to start is by identifying your vague discontent, that phenomenon that "bugs" you, that you want an explanation for: your "concept of concern." Call it whatever it appears to you to be, and then begin your exploration—through the literature, through your own experience and that of others.* Intuition plays a large part in this process, both in the relationships you choose to look at and in the search through the literature. The influence of intuition on the review of the literature is the reason computer searches are not totally

---

*Norris' article describing her exploration of the concept of restlessness is a good example of this process.[13]

reliable. They are not programmed to lead you *off* the beaten track to that crazy little study which somehow gives you the "aha" you have been looking for.

But intuition will of necessity be subjected to orderly criticism, and the more explicit one is about the hunches which go into the development of a theoretical framework, the easier it is to subject those hunches to testing and thereby strengthen the theoretical base.

When one is clear about one's concept of concern, it is necessary to do a very thorough review of the literature in order to identify as many of the factors which are related to the concept as possible. Blalock calls this process an inventory of causes and effects. In order to avoid causal terminology, it may be thought of as an inventory of related factors. Nevertheless, it is necessary to specify the direction of the relationships (refer to Chapter 2), i.e., whether A leads to B or vice versa. At this point in the review it is also important to very carefully evaluate the validity of the reported relationships. Inevitably there will be conflicting findings, and ultimately one will have to reconcile the contradictions. The inventory of related factors will begin something like this (Fig. 6):

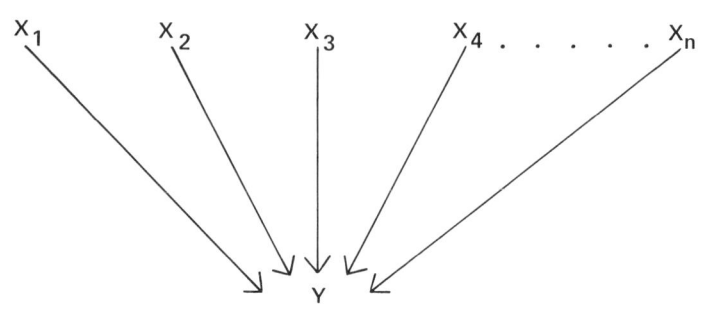

FIGURE 6. Inventory of related factors.

PROCESS OF SYNTHESIZING A THEORY

Let Y represent the focal concept (your "concept of concern") and the X's the possible explanation for the phenomenon. Eventually the diagram should be expanded to include the "effects" of Y, but initially it is enough to deal with the factors that have been demonstrated to relate to changes in Y. Each one of the $X \to Y$ relationships represents a proposition or law of interrelationship.

The following exposition is my attempt to illustrate this process from my own pursuit of a theory of time perception. Initially, my vague discontent derived from patients' complaints of "time dragging." At the same time, the concept of time perception appealed to me as a holistic indicator of health status; therefore the concept met certain criteria that were important to me: it was consistent with the conceptual framework within which I had chosen to work, and it represented a realistic problem of people identified as patients. The next step then was to review the literature, state the propositions, and diagram the related factors. In this process, it became apparent that time perception is a rather global term which includes many subconcepts, and the aspect in which I was most interested was perception of duration; therefore my inventory was limited to this concept. The initial inventory is shown in Figure 7.

At this point, the X factors are considered to be independent of each other, even though in reality they are not. Another level of abstraction is needed in order for the diagram to have any meaning or explanatory value. The question one must ask is:

> Are there similarities among the X factors that would give some clue as to why or how they influence the Y factor?

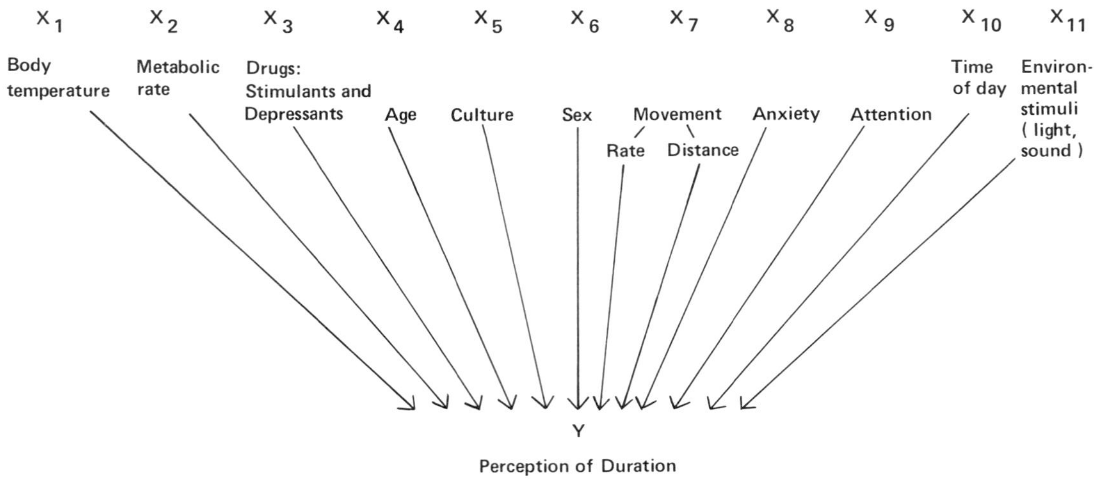

FIGURE 7. Initial inventory of related factors (Newman, 1971).

PROCESS OF SYNTHESIZING A THEORY

From Figure 7 it can be seen that a number of the X factors in the inventory of relationships are related to a change in rate of biological activity: body temperature, metabolic rate, and drugs.[14] Moreover, the idea of activity rate as an explanation for perceived duration extends into the psychological realm in that emotional state and amount of attention paid to a task are related to the number of events of which the individual is aware. Therefore I specified biological event rate (I_1) and psychological event rate (I_2) as the intervening variables[14] (see Fig. 8).*

If the intervening variables are sufficient, then all factors influencing perception of duration should be mediated through them.† As already suggested, one can start with the isolated factors and, based on similarities, conceptualize the intervening variables, or one may begin with the summary concepts and deduce factors which apply to the phenomenon in question.

Somewhere in the process of reviewing the literature and examining the relationships, I settled on the relationship which I wanted to test: body movement and perceived duration. Does movement fit the conceptualization posed? Certainly movement is a factor in rate of biological activity, and it can be a factor in rate of psychological

---

*In order to simplify the diagram, I have removed the environmental and demographic factors which can be controlled in the research design.

---

†Blalock[6] cites a clearer example of intervening variables in relation to population change. He asserts that all factors influencing population change will be subsets of deaths, births, immigration, and emigration.

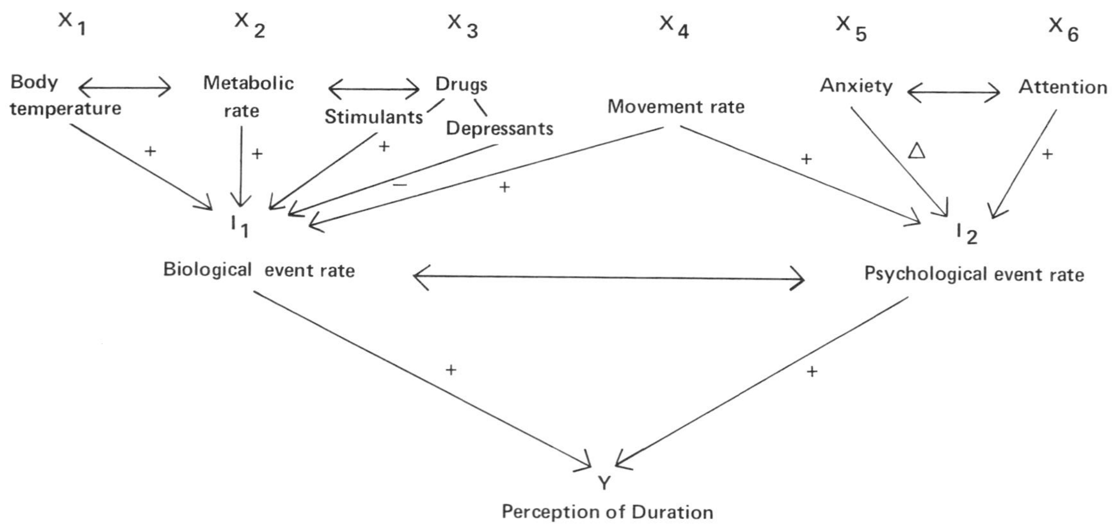

FIGURE 8. Revised inventory of related factors, specifying intervening variables (Newman, 1971).

PROCESS OF SYNTHESIZING A THEORY

activity (as when one becomes aware of every step taken). The axioms at this stage of the development of the theory were as follows:

1. An increase in the rate of biological events will produce a relative increase in perceived duration.
2. An increase in discrete events of which one is aware will produce a relative increase in perceived duration.
3. An increase in the rate of movement will produce an increase in rate of biological events.
4. An increase in the rate of movement will produce an increase in the number of discrete events of which one is aware.

Figure 9 represents a diagram of these axioms.

Therefore the theorem to be tested is:

Rate of movement will be directly related to perceived duration.

Even though the axioms are stated in causal terms in order to make explicit the direction of the relationship, the derived theorem is stated as a relationship because it is to be tested, and one cannot test causality.

The first set of axioms in the development of theory will undoubtedly omit many important factors. Such was the case of the above formulation: the results of the testing of this theorem did not support the relationship.[15] The study did reveal a factor which was omitted from the set of axioms and which appeared to be an important factor in influencing the results. Subjects reported their conscious

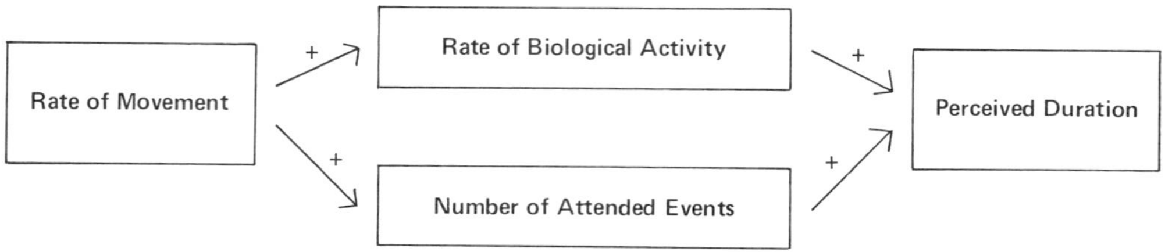

FIGURE 9. Diagram of Newman's axioms (1971).

PROCESS OF SYNTHESIZING A THEORY

efforts to compensate for the effect of the rate of movement on their judgment of time. The following propositions then had to be incorporated in the set of axioms:

> Time perception is a function of a learned relationship between movement and clock time.
>
> If rate of movement changes from an individual's preferred rate of movement, he will consciously compensate for this change in order to judge time according to his usual gauge.

The oversight in Figure 9 reflects a view of man as simply the passive recipient of the biological and psychological events imposed upon him. Recognizing that in the processing of the stimuli which he is receiving, both from within and without, he interacts with the stimuli, one sees that the model must incorporate the interaction of event rate and conscious compensation in order to reflect more accurately the man-environment interaction which was an assumption of the conceptual framework but was overlooked in the zeal of condensing the theory. The question now is: Will the movement → perceived duration relationship manifest itself if conscious compensation can be controlled? That represented the next stage of testing.

The more I struggled with the conceptualization of the intervening variables through which events are interpreted in terms of the passage of time, the more I came to the conclusion that perceived duration is a function of the relationship of awareness of events to content of events (see Fig. 10). This conceptualization is similar to Ornstein's[16] approach, which states that perceived duration is a func-

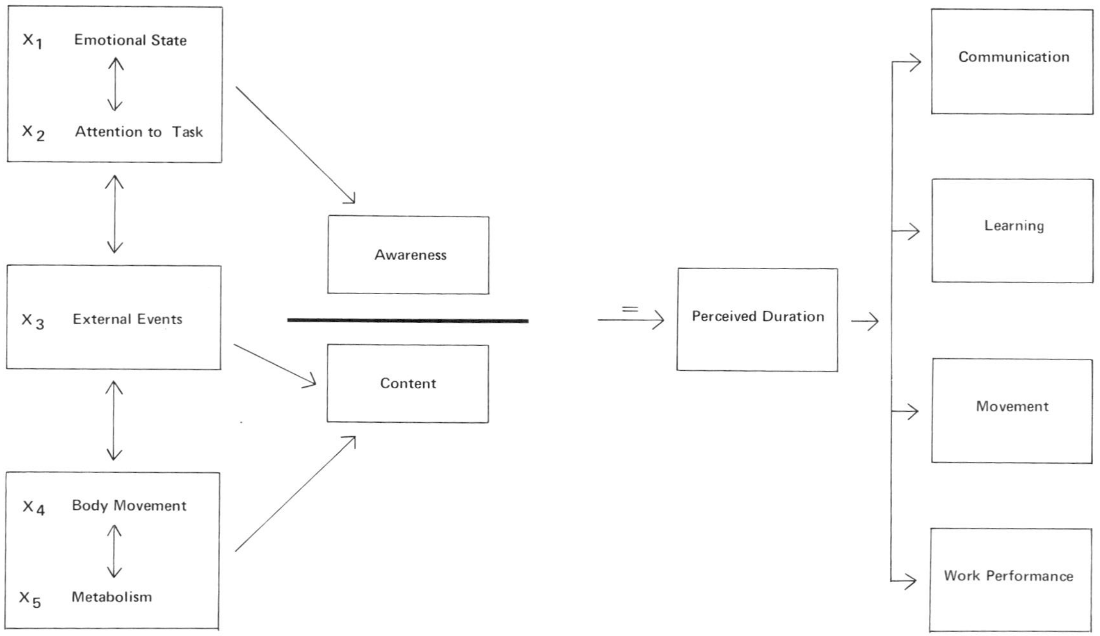

FIGURE 10. Revised diagram of Newman's axioms.

PROCESS OF SYNTHESIZING A THEORY

tion of the amount and organization of the units of information processing.

One can then begin to speculate as to which specific factors would make a difference in the major consolidations, represented by the boxes on the left hand side of Figure 10. These consolidated factors, in turn, influence the ratio of awareness to content. An example of how this would work would be an instance of heightened awareness and low content. This would result in a change of perceived duration in the direction of overestimation.

The righthand column of boxes represents an inventory of "effects," as mentioned earlier in the chapter. When one begins to be satisfied with the intervening variables which offer some explanation of the phenomenon of concern, the next phase is to begin to examine the relationship of that phenomenon to health, and in Figure 10, I have speculated as to what factors may be influenced by one's awareness of time.

This diagram represents a theory in progress. Theory, in order to be nursing theory, must go beyond describing, explaining, and predicting a particular phenomenon. It must specify and test the actions necessary in order to promote health, the stated purpose in nursing. Therefore, every theory must extend beyond the explanation of the phenomenon to an explanation of its specific relationship to health.

6

TOWARD A THEORY OF HEALTH

Current conceptual models in nursing emphasize the focus of the nursing process, i.e., the phenomenon of man, or the interactive component, which facilitates that process. Although most nursing theorists recognize health as the goal of nursing, the terms used to define health are often broad and general and are subject to multiple interpretations. A precise conceptualization of the nature of health is required in order to specify theory which relates to that phenomenon.

Most would agree that health is *not* the absence of disease, or complete psychological and social well-being, for these states are nonexistent in the complexity of our changing world. Some progress was made in an understanding of health when health and illness were placed on a continuum. This conceptualization recognizes the dynamic, changing relationships portraying different degrees of health and illness; however, it still maintains the dichotomy between the two by polarizing health at one end of the continuum and illness at the other end. If the goal of nursing is to move the individual toward health, then in this context, that means *away* from illness. In so doing, the dichotomy is maintained.

What is needed is a synthesis of the concepts of health and illness. This view is based on Hegel's dialectical process of the fusion of opposites: one state of being unites with its opposite and brings forth a synthesis of the two. Applying this process to health and illness, there is, on the one hand, a condition specified as disease and, on the other hand, its opposite, which will be called non-disease. The fusion of the two antithetical concepts brings forth a synthesis, which can be regarded as health.

$$\text{Disease—Non-disease} \rightarrow \text{Health}$$

When health is viewed as the synthesis of disease and non-disease, the following statements can be considered as basic assumptions:

1. *Health encompasses conditions heretofore described as illness, or in medical terms, pathology.*
   A person who has a pathological condition is not necessarily "ill." Experience with persons incapacitated in various ways by chronic disease reveals that, for the most part, these people do not consider themselves sick. They may be unable to walk or to care for themselves, but from their point of view, they are *not* sick, unless perhaps they are inconvenienced by the common cold. As a matter of fact, nearly everyone of adult age has some condition which could be specified as pathological, with varying degrees of in-

capacitation, but each person is still very much a whole person.

2. *These "pathological" conditions can be considered a manifestation of the total pattern of the individual.*
This statement is based on Rogers' prior assumption that "Pattern and organization identify man and reflect his innovative wholeness" [p. 65].[9] The pattern which is manifested in disease may be regarded as a clue to what is going on in the person's life, the dynamics of which the person may be unaware of and cannot communicate in any other way.

3. *The pattern of the individual that eventually manifests itself as pathology is primary and exists prior to structural or functional changes.*
An illustration of this point may be seen in Bahnson and Bahnson's[17] theory regarding the rhythms of cancer. They maintain that the person who develops cancer manifests a pattern of very controlled interaction with the environment and very uncontrolled or chaotic internal processes; another way of describing it would be as rigid external rhythms and disorganized internal rhythms. If this theory holds, the pattern exists prior to the development of the cancer; the cancer is simply a manifestation of the pattern.

4. *Removal of the pathology in itself will not change the pattern of the individual.*
This principle can be seen in the previous example regarding cancer. The pattern of which the cancer is a manifestation is a total pattern of the person. Removal of the cancer will not change the basic pattern. As Western medicine has begun to seek holistic approaches, practitioners are beginning to recognize

that disease is not something "to be gotten rid of," but something to be understood and experienced and regarded as a teacher or message. Disease can be regarded as an integrating factor, and as such, it is important in the evolutionary process of the individual, and not something to be squelched.

5. *If becoming "ill" is the only way an individual's pattern can manifest itself, then that is health for that person.*

Illness, as an integrating factor, may accomplish for the person what he was unable to do otherwise. Stone,[18] a Jungian psychologist who has embraced a holistic approach to health and illness, points out that in his practice he "doesn't keep track of people getting well anymore." Not that he is not pleased when someone does "get well," and not that feeling well is an unimportant consideration, but it is not of such importance that it is sought to the exclusion of the higher purpose of integration of self, which then frees energy for an expanding consciousness.

6. *Health is the expansion of consciousness.*

Health is viewed as the totality of the life process, which is evolving toward expanded consciousness. Man represents one stage of this evolution. The direction of evolution within the individual person as well as within the species of mankind is toward expansion of awareness to greater dimensions.

CONCEPTUAL FRAMEWORK

Based on this synthesized view of health, what are the basic concepts the interrelations of which describe the

TOWARD A THEORY OF HEALTH

process? Any attempt to identify and understand the basic components of such a process might be considered a presumptuous endeavor. Capra,[19] a physicist, points out that a current hypothesis in physics "not only denies the existence of fundamental constituents of matter, but accepts no fundamental entities whatsoever—no fundamental laws, equations, or principles." Such a position, however, does not preclude an attempt to understand the total by an examination of selected phenomena. He continues:

> Physicists have come to see that all their theories of natural phenomena, including the 'laws' they describe, are creations of the human mind; properties of our conceptual map of reality, rather than reality itself. The conceptual scheme is necessarily limited and approximate, as are all the scientific theories and 'laws of nature' it contains. All natural phenomena are ultimately interconnected, and in order to explain any one of them we need to understand all the others, which is obviously impossible. What makes science so successful is the discovery that approximations are possible. If one is satisfied with an approximate 'understanding' of nature, one can describe selected groups of phenomena in this way, neglecting other phenomena which are less relevant. Thus one can explain many phenomena in terms of a few, and consequently understand different aspects of nature in an approximate way without having to understand everything at once.

That is the intent in this conceptual framework: to understand many phenomena, the phenomena of the life process, and therefore of health, in terms of a few. The concepts which constitute this framework are movement, time, space, and consciousness.

```
           Consciousness
                /\
               /  \
              /    \
Movement <---/------\---> Space
             \      /
              \    /
               \  /
               Time
```

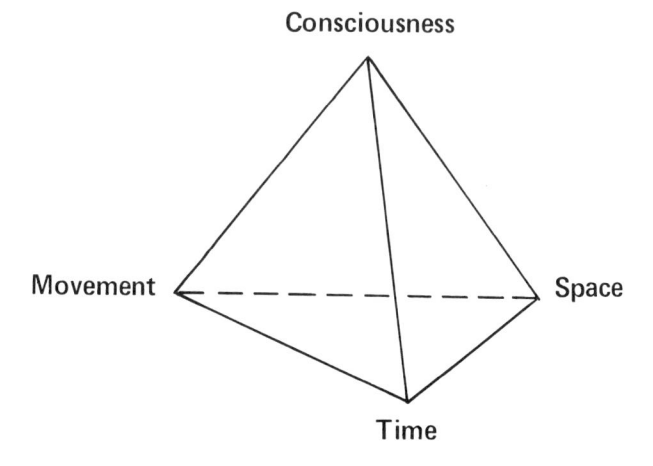

The postulated interrelationships of these concepts are as follows:

1. Time and space have a complementary relationship.
2. Movement is a means whereby space and time become a reality.
3. Movement is a reflection of consciousness.
4. Time is a function of movement.
5. Time is a measure of consciousness.

Life, as we know it, is composed of the energy of matter and motion, and each may be transformed into the other. The energy of motion is transformed into the energy of mass, and vice versa. At the subatomic level, particles have no meaning as isolated entities but only as interconnections of things. The world, then, must be viewed as a complicated network of interrelated changing events, as dynamic patterns of activity, with space aspects and time aspects.[19]

TOWARD A THEORY OF HEALTH

The complementarity of space and time can be seen at different levels of analysis. At the level of macrocosmic systems there is the likelihood of antimatter galaxies where time flows in the opposite direction from our perspective, and "black holes" in space where time and space are "wrapped up" by gravitation in unimaginable ways; at the microcosmic level, subatomic particles of matter appear to be going backward in time.[20] The complementarity of space and time can also be seen in everyday events. The highly mobile individual lives in a world of expanded space and compartmentalized time. When one's life space is decreased, as by either physical or social immobility, one's time is increased. Such a situation can be an opportunity for attention to the space that is within. As one is able to transcend the limitation of three-dimensional space, the experience of time changes and with it the level of consciousness. The concept of space, then, is inextricably linked to the concept of time. There is reason to believe that the nature of the relationship which is being described at the macrocosmic and microcosmic levels will hold also at the humanistic level as the concepts of life space, personal space, and inner space are examined in relation to time.

Movement is an essential property of matter. Movement brings about change, without which there is no manifest reality. The reality of our world is manifest in the change occurring between two states of rest.[21] This action-rest cycle is evident at the micro level in nerve action spikes and complex muscular rhythms, and at the macro level in the pattern of body movements, breathing rhythms, and interactive patterns of life activities. Illustrating this action-rest cycle, the pattern of body movement contains the necessary rhythm of preparation, action, and recovery.[22]

Within this general pattern, the body movement of each person is specific to that person. Each individual naturally adopts a walking tempo which is most efficient in energy expenditure for that person.[23] The total pattern of movement appears to be reflective of the organization or disorganization of the thought and feeling processes of the individual. Disharmony in the body-world system is reflected in disharmony of body movements. Where there is excess tension, this leads to alienation of the affected parts of the body, and there is loss of versatility of potential action. Action requires internal organization as well as clarity of organization of the corresponding world structure. Changes in either internal organization or perception of external organization will be reflected in the pattern of movement.[22]

Movement is seen, then, as an awareness of self. Awareness of self is closely connected with awareness of the body. Kinesthetic awareness is viewed by some as the "basic process of knowing which subtends all bodily actions, and synthesizes them."[24] Further it is considered to be the basic perceptual organ of space and time as it contains memory of the past and expectations of the future. For instance, when we become angry or hurt, these feelings are reflected in our muscles and may remain there unless released through aggressive action. The muscles become a kind of storehouse for locked energies. In addition, our world space is changed each time we make a move; the objects of the world are perceived in terms of their potential movements, or the possibilities for action.[22]

Movement is a means of communicating. We express ourselves in movement and gesture. This expression of self in movement is refined in the body arts, but occurs more generally on a day-to-day basis. Language itself requires a rhythm of muscular activity, which consists of successive waves of patterned movements. This rhythm is shared by the listener. The harmony of the movement-speech configuration of the speaker is reflected in the muscular patterns of the listener, provided that they are relating: "This mutual dance facilitates an empathic understanding of the other person's world through complementary movements."[22] The rhythm and pattern which are reflected in movement are an indication of the internal organization of the person and his perception of the world. Movement provides a means of communication beyond that which language can convey.

Movement relates also to the experience of time. The illusiveness of time has been a mystery which has intrigued philosophers for centuries. Einstein's theory of relativity brought the relativity and subjectivity of the time experience under scrutiny by the scientific community, and subsequently scientists in nearly every field have sought to describe and understand the meaning of time. Piaget,[25] in his studies of both children and adults, led the way in postulating time as a function of movement. This relationship is supported by my previous research, e.g., when an individual is forced to walk at a rate which is slower than his perferred rate of walking (normal tempo), his perception of time changes.[15,26] The slower one walks, the faster the objective time of the world seems to be passing. (This relationship seems to be modified by the individual's awareness of the movement activity, as described in the previous chapter.)

In addition to the relationship between movement and time, an even more intriguing association seems to be emerging from these data: a relationship between age and time. On the surface, this relationship appears to contradict the movement-time nexus, since from a number of standpoints, the older person appears to be slowing down. If this were true, extrapolating from the movement-time relationship, one would anticipate that time would be perceived as passing faster. The opposite appears to be true on preliminary testing; another explanation is needed.

Bentov[27] has postulated that time is a measure of consciousness. He calculates an index of consciousness by establishing a ratio of subjective time (the number of seconds judged to have elapsed) to objective time (actual clock time). For example, if one thinks 4 seconds have elapsed, but according to the clock, only 1 second has elapsed, the ratio would be 4/1 with a resulting index of consciousness of 4 (as compared to a ratio of $1/1 = 1$). When this index is applied to the data from my previous research,[15,26] it reveals the following trend:

Age (Means)	Time Subjective/ Objective		Consciousness Index
23 (N=52)	40/43	=	.93
28 (N=90)	40/31	=	1.29
71 (N=23)	40/17	=	2.35

With increasing age, the index of consciousness increases. These data are consistent with the position that the direction of the life process is toward expansion of consciousness.

In recent years, studies of the brain have made us aware that there are dimensions of consciousness which have

TOWARD A THEORY OF HEALTH

been neglected and, to some extent, have not been easily available to us. The major hemisphere, usually the left, is primarily responsible for the analytical, sequence-perceiving processes, while the minor hemisphere, usually the right, is primarily responsible for the synthesis-oriented, symbolic and intuitive modes. The scientific and technological values of our Western society have emphasized the rational, logical processes to the neglect of intuitive, holistic processes. This emphasis has been reinforced developmentally, in that processing in one hemisphere inhibits processes in the other.[28] With the recognition that the products of logical rational approaches are not necessarily desirable, we have begun to recognize the need for the development and facilitation of the intuitive processes. We have available to us a realm of consciousness which many of us are not utilizing. This situation can be likened to tuning in to a small AM radio rather than a refined stereophonic system. The possibility exists for us to tune in to higher frequencies. The human range of frequency response extends into the astral realm. According to Bentov,[27] the fact that some human beings are able to perceive at the higher end of this range explains the experiences of so-called paranormal, or psychic, phenomena. The direction of the evolution of life is toward higher and greater frequency of energy exchange.

As the process of evolution takes place, we must be prepared for, and recognize in others, jumps in consciousness beyond our present capacities. Scholars from a variety of disciplines are in agreement that there is no matter devoid of consciousness and that consciousness is coextensive.[29,30,31] The higher the level of consciousness, the more the interpenetration of energy fields, and with this interpenetration, evolutionary jumps occur. According to Bentov,[21] you "catch it [expanded consciousness] like you catch the flu." Watson[29] illustrates this point with an example from studies of monkey colonies on a small island adjacent to the southernmost island of Japan. In 1952 the winter was particularly severe, and the monkeys were given supplementary feedings of sweet potatoes. There was a problem, however, with the containers for the food, and the potatoes fell out and became coated with sand, which made it difficult for the moneys to eat them. One day a young female monkey took her sweet potato to a nearby freshwater stream and washed it. According to Watson, such an innovation in the monkey world was "tantamount to inventing the wheel." This young monkey then taught her mother and her siblings and her other monkey friends how to wash the potatoes. Very slowly the knowledge spread through the community of monkeys. Six years passed, and in March 1957, a significant number of monkeys, perhaps 99 in all, had learned to wash potatoes. Then the hundredth monkey learned the trick, and 20 minutes later every monkey in the community was doing it! By that evening monkeys on two neighboring islands, with no physical contact, were washing sweet potatoes! The knowledge had reached a kind of critical threshold, or critical mass, beyond which it became common knowledge.

SUMMARY

The expansion of consciousness is what life, and therefore health, is all about. Movement, time, and space have been selected as correlates of developing consciousness and means whereby we can gain some understanding of the process. This framework provides a view of health as the totality of life process and therefore one which encompasses disease as a meaningful aspect. In this context, the goal of nursing is not to make people well, or to prevent their getting sick, but to assist people to utilize the power that is within them as they evolve toward higher levels of consciousness.

7

SEARCHING FOR MORE HOLISTIC METHODS OF INQUIRY

As relative newcomers to the field of scientific inquiry, nursing researchers have adopted predominantly the methodology of other disciplines in pursuit of nursing knowledge. But just as social scientists have recognized that the methods of physical science could not totally satisfy their needs, so also nursing scientists are discovering that the methods of traditional science may not be sufficent for their needs. It is questionable, for instance, whether or not the phenomena being measured in much of nursing research are really manifestations of wholeness. Furthermore, how can measurement at one point in time (if indeed that is possible) reflect the dynamic nature of the phenomena? As nursing scientists become increasingly sophisticated in methodology and confident in the focus of nursing inquiry, there is a need to develop methods which will depict the holistic, dynamic nature of man as a living system in a constantly changing world. Moreover, there is a need to keep in mind the ultimate purpose of theory development in nursing and to utilize methods which are reflective of the complexity of the real-world situation of practitioner and client.

A holistic approach is not to be confused with, or construed to mean, a multivariate approach. It is not the summing up of many factors (psychological, social, physiological, and so on) to make a whole. It is the identification of patterns which are reflective of the whole. What these parameters are will vary according to one's ability to see the whole. For some, the universe can be seen in a grain of sand. For others, characteristics which present identifiable patterns of the individual, e.g., the way a person walks or the way he talks, are a good place to start. The task is not easy. When one has grasped the meaning of holism and identified the phenomenon of inquiry, the next step is to find valid ways of measuring it.

Maslow[32] has suggested that in the study of human problems we begin with a phenomenological approach. Basic to such an approach is the need for researchers to be astute observers, or as Maslow put it more cogently, "good knowers." In our zeal to obtain valid and reliable research instruments, we may have overlooked the most sensitive of all instruments to measure another human being—ourselves. As we become more knowledgeable about intuition and the powers of our consciousness, we are aware that there is more to knowing than that which we obtain by rational, analytic methods.

Another problem is that much of the research thus far in nursing does not get at intraindividual change, and therefore, can offer no information regarding intraindividual patterns or trends. The majority of the designs have been one-shot comparisons of characteristics within a specific population or cross-sectional designs of a particular characteristic in different age groups. The data are reported in group averages, and, in the case of cross-sectional designs, an assumption must be made that the age groups are from the same population, when we know in reality that there are generational differences. Since, at least at this stage of nursing's knowledge, we need to be able to identify changing intraindividual patterns, it may well be that we will learn more by taking a closer look at fewer cases over time than by looking at many cases at one time. Certainly, much of the research on rhythmic phenomena requires such an approach. As we become clearer as to what phenomena need to be measured and how to measure them, we can then utilize more complex designs which incorporate both longitudinal and cross-sectional testing and thus provide information about intraindividual change in a changing world.[33]

Susman and Evered,[34] scientists in the field of administrative theory, are particularly concerned about the inadequacies of the more traditional, rationalistic methods of science in the development of theories of practice. Their explication of action research as a method for developing theories of practice within living, open systems seems particularly applicable to the need for theories of practice within nursing.

Action research involves the collaboration of the researcher in the real-world situation of the client system with the purposes of improving the situation, developing the competencies of the system, and generating new knowledge. In terms of nursing, the client system would be composed of the nursing practitioner and the client. The purpose of the process would be to improve the health of the client, develop the competencies of the practitioner, and generate new nursing knowledge. The cyclical nature of the process would be the same as that described by Susman and Evered: diagnostic planning, action-taking, data-gathering, evaluative interpreting, and specifying learnings.

Although the aim of action research is the development of prescriptive-level theory, the method itself is not simply the application and testing of a pre-existing prescriptive solution. It is a continuous collaborative experience with practitioners as the problem is identified and actions are taken to resolve the problem. The situation-problem-action nexus is under continuous revision. Whereas with traditional methods, the problem and solutions are determined in advance and imposed upon a situation, in action research, the researcher begins by being unclear about the situation, problem and actions, and must collaborate with the practitioner and work within a living system. The researcher recognizes that every situation is unique and that the outcome of selected actions cannot be fully known in advance; the process is continuously exploratory in nature.

Susman and Evered assert that action research can make the following contributions to the growth of knowledge:

1. The development of action principles dealing with situational diversity.
2. The development of new kinds of technologies, such as how to diagnose and how to do something that is *not* prescribed.
3. The development of action competencies—the types of skills needed by practitioners, such as interpretation and judgment skills.

MORE HOLISTIC METHODS OF INQUIRY

4. The development of the researchers' own competencies of how to act in unprescribed situations.

All of the above outcomes are pertinent to the need in nursing for theories of practice. One further aspect of action research which seems particularly relevant is that it necessitates increased contact and authentic collaboration between the researchers and practitioners. The results of such collaboration should increase the relevance of research to practice and facilitate the application of findings.

Nursing has made considerable progress during the past quarter of a century toward the development of nursing science. We, along with scientists in other disciplines, are on the forefront of exciting new discoveries regarding the development of man and how this relates to health. Scientists from each discipline see these discoveries as an expansion of their own discipline: physicists see it as the expansion of physics, psychologists see it as within their realm, and so on. The same is true regarding the practice which is based on that knowledge. The medical profession sees holistic health as its "rightful heritage," while psychologists have moved ahead in this arena, making contributions of their own. From my standpoint as a nursing scientist, I see the expansion of knowledge related to man's health and the development of practice based on that knowledge as the responsibility, and perhaps the "rightful heritage," of nursing.

We now have a relatively clear concept of the phenomenon of our inquiry. This movement toward a central focus represents, not a unified theory of nursing, but rather an agreement as to what it is we must understand in order to practice nursing. Various conceptual frameworks centered on man as a living system in interaction with a changing environment have emerged, providing the basis for multiple theories regarding health. Nursing theory, then, is theory which describes, explains, and predicts the patterns of the life process of man which are conducive to health and which prescribes actions to promote these patterns. This type of knowledge requires methodologies compatible with the dynamic nature of the phenomena and the complexity of nursing practice.

REFERENCES

1. Nightingale, Florence: *Notes on Nursing: What It Is, and What It Is Not*. Harrison, London, 1859 (facsimile ed., J.B. Lippincott, Philadelphia, 1957; paperback ed., Dover, New York, 1969).
2. Dickoff, James, and James, Patricia: *Theory of theories: a position paper*. Nurs. Res. 17:197–203, 1968.
3. Hempel, Carl G.: *Fundamentals of Concept Formation in Empirical Science*. University of Chicago Press, Chicago, 1952.
4. Popper, Karl R.: *Conjectures and Refutations: The Growth of Scientific Knowledge*. Harper & Row, New York, 1968.
5. Dubin, Robert: *Theory Building*. The Free Press, New York, 1978.
6. Blalock, Hubert M., Jr.: *Theory Construction: From Verbal to Mathematical Formulations*. Prentice-Hall, Englewood Cliffs, New Jersey, 1969.
7. Johnson, Dorothy E.: *One conceptual model of nursing*. Unpublished paper presented at Vanderbilt University, Nashville, Tennessee, April 25, 1968.

8. Roy, Sr. Callista: *The Roy adaptation model*, in Riehl, Joan P., and Roy, Sr. Callista (eds.): *Conceptual Models for Nursing Practice.* Appleton-Century-Crofts, New York, 1974.
9. Rogers, Martha E.: *An Introduction to the Theoretical Basis of Nursing.* F.A. Davis, Philadelphia, 1970.
10. Grubbs, Judy: *The Johnson behavioral system model*, in Riehl, Joan P., and Roy, Sr. Callista (eds.): *Conceptual Models for Nursing Practice.* Appleton-Centrury-Crofts, New York, 1974.
11. Schlachter, Louise: *The Relation Between Anxiety, Perceived Body and Personal Space, and Actual Body Space Among Young Female Adults.* Unpublished Ph.D. dissertation, New York University, 1971.
12. Rodgers, Janet A.: *The Relationship Between Sociability and Personal Space Preferences Among College Students in the Morning and in the Afternoon.* Unpublished Ph.D. dissertation, New York University, 1971.
13. Norris, Catherine M.: *Restlessness: a phenomenon in search of meaning.* Nurs. Outlook 23:103–107, 1975.
14. Newman, Margaret A.: *An Investigation of the Relationship Between Gait Tempo and Time Perception.* Unpublished Ph.D. dissertation, New York University, 1971.
15. Newman, Margaret A.: *Time estimation in relation to gait tempo.* Percept. Motor Skills 34:359–366, 1972.
16. Ornstein, Robert E.: *On the Experience of Time.* Penguin Books, Baltimore, 1969.
17. Bahnson, C.B., and Bahnson, M.B.: *Role of the ego defenses: denial and repression in the etiology of malignant neoplasm.* Ann. N.Y. Acad. Sci. 125(3):827–845, 1966.
18. Stone, Harold: *Holism: a new vision of man, a new vision of health.* Paper presented at conference on Holistic Perspectives: A Renaissance in Medicine and Health Care, Philadelphia, November 11–12, 1978.

REFERENCES

19. Capra, Fritjof: *The Tao of Physics*. Shambhala Publications, Boulder, Colorado, 1975.
20. Pelletier, Kenneth R.: *Toward a Science of Consciousness*. Dell, New York, 1978, p. 56.
21. Bentov, Itzhak: *The mechanics of consciousness*. Paper presented at symposium on New Dimensions of Consciousness, sponsored by Sufi Order in the West, New York, November 17–20, 1978.
22. Hall, R.L., and Cobey, V.E.: *The world of crystallized movement*. Main Currents 31(1):4–7, September-October 1974.
23. Ralston, J.H.: *Energy-speed relation and optimal speed during level walking*. Int. Z. Angewandte Physiol. Einsch. Arbeitsphysiol. 17:277, 1958.
24. Mickunas, Algis: *The primacy of movement*. Main Currents 31(1):8–12, September–October 1974.
25. Piaget, Jean: *Time perception in children*, in Fraser, J.T. (ed.): *The Voices of Time*. George Braziller, New York, 1966.
26. Newman, Margaret A.: *Movement tempo and the experience of time*. Nurs. Res. 25:273–279, 1976.
27. Bentov, Itzhak: *Stalking the Wild Pendulum*. E.P. Dutton, New York, 1977.
28. Fischer, Roland, and Rhead, John: *The logical and the intuitive*. Main Currents 31(2):50–54, November–December 1974.
29. Watson, Lyall: *Evolution and the unconscious*. Paper presented at symposium on New Dimensions of Consciousness, sponsored by Sufi Order in the West, New York, November 17–20, 1978.
30. Capra, Fritjof: *The Tao of physics*. Paper presented at symposium on New Dimensions of Consciousness, sponsored by Sufi Order in the West, New York, November 17–20, 1978.

31. Muses, Charles: *Higher dimensions and systems relating science and spirit*. Paper presented at symposium on New Dimensions of Consciousness, sponsored by Sufi Order in the West, New York, November 17–20, 1978.
32. Maslow, Abraham H.: *The Psychology of Science*. Harper & Row, New York, 1966.
33. Baltes, Paul B., Reese, Hayne W., and Nesselroade, John: *Life-Span Development Psychology: Introduction to Research Method*. Wadsworth, Belmont, California, 1977.
34. Susman, Gerald I., and Evered, Roger D.: *An assessment of the scientific merits of action research*. Admin. Sci. Q. 23:582–603, December 1978.

APPENDICES

Appendix A

Basic Components of the Nursing Conceptual Models of Johnson, Roy, and Rogers*

	Johnson	Roy	Rogers
Focus	Views man as a behavioral system composed of interrelated parts and elements of behavior (subsystems).	Views man as a biopsychosocial being.	Views man as a unified whole possessing his own integrity and manifesting characteristics that are more than and different from the sum of his parts.
Basic Assumptions	The patterned and repetitive ways of behaving that characterize the life of man are conceived as forming an organized and integrating whole.		The unidirectionality of life proceeds rhythmically along a spiral, revealing cyclical continuity. What seems to be repetition is, in reality, only similarity. The continuous change ... is expressed in the continuing emergence of new patterns in man and environment.

Man strives continually to maintain a behavioral system balance, a steady state, by more or less automatic adjustments and adaptations to the "natural" forces impinging upon him.

Behavioral system balance is essential to man... [and] reflects adjustment or adaptation which is "successful" in some way or to some degree....

Man seeks new experiences which may disturb his steady state temporarily and which may require behavioral modifications to reestablish balance.

Man is in constant interaction with a changing environment... To cope with a changing world, man uses both innate and acquired mechanisms, which are biological, psychologic, and social in origin.

To respond positively to environmental changes, man must adapt.

Man's capacity to maintain himself while undergoing continuous change is a remarkable characteristic... Commonly referred to as man's self-regulating ability... Directed toward achieving increasing complexity of organization — not toward achieving equilibrium and stability.

Man is represented as... becoming increasingly complex [and]... evolving rhythmically. Pattern and organization are maintained amidst the constant change attending the continuous interaction between man and environment.

Appendix A. *Continued.*

	Johnson	Roy	Rogers
	Man's behavioral responses are developed and modified over time through maturation and experience; they are determined developmentally and are continuously governed by a multitude of biological, psychological, and social factors operating in a complex and interlocking fashion.	Man's adaptation is a function of the stimulus he is exposed to and his adaptation level (determined by focal, contextual, and residual stimuli).	Change in the human field depends only upon the state of the human field and the simultaneous state of the environmental field at any given point in space-time.
Purpose (Goal) of Nursing	... is thought to be that of behavioral system equilibrium and dynamic stability. ... nursing's specific contribution to patient welfare is that of fostering efficient and effective behavioral functioning in the patient to prevent illness and during and following illness.	To bring about an adapted state in the patient which frees him to respond to other stimuli which may be present.	... seeks to promote symphonic interaction between man and environment, to strengthen the coherence and integrity of the human field, and to direct and redirect patterning of the human and environmental fields for realization of maximum health potential.

Health and Illness	Health and illness are one inevitable dimension of man's life—viewed as a continuum from very healthy to very ill.	Health and sickness are expressions of the process of life. Their meaning is derived out of an understanding of the life process in its totality.
Definition of Nursing	... an external regulatory force which acts to preserve the organization and integration of the patient's behavior under those conditions in which illness is found.	... focuses on human being—on man in his entirety and wholeness.
	... focuses on the patient as a person adapting to those stimuli present as a result of his position on the health-illness continuum.	... encompasses the man-environment relationship and seeks to identify sequential, cross-sectional patterning in the life process.
		... is directed toward repatterning of man and environment for more effective fulfillment of life's capabilities.

Appendix A. Continued.

	Johnson	Roy	Rogers
Basis for Assessment	Extent to which patient has attained the goals of the behavioral subsystems: achievement, affiliative, aggressive/protective, dependency, eliminative, ingestive, restorative, sexual.	Extent to which patient has achieved an adapted state within the four adaptive modes: physiologic, self-concept, role function, interdependence.	Identification of sequential, cross-sectional patterning in the life process: total configuration; nature, amount, and speed of wave propagation which leads to enhancement or disruption of man's environment.

*Material included in this comparison has been excerpted and adapted from the following sources:

Grubbs, Judy: *The Johnson behavioral system model*, in Riehl, Joan P., and Roy, Sr. Callista (eds.): *Conceptual Models for Nursing Practice*. Appleton-Century-Crofts, New York, 1974, pp. 160–197.

Johnson, Dorothy E.: *One conceptual model of nursing*. Unpublished paper presented at Vanderbilt University, Nashville, Tennessee, April 25, 1968.

Rogers, Martha E.: *An Introduction to the Theoretical Basis of Nursing*. F.A. Davis, Philadelphia, 1970.

Roy, Sr. Callista: *The Roy adaptation model*, in Riehl, Joan P., and Roy, Sr. Callista (eds.): *Conceptual Models for Nursing Practice*. Appleton-Century-Crofts, New York, 1974, pp. 135–144.

Appendix B

Definitions of Constructs and Statements of Hypotheses from Schlachter's Study

Anxiety: Apprehension initiated by a threat to those values necessary for the preservation of the individual's personality, as measured by the IPAT Anxiety Scale by Cattell and Scheier.

Perceived personal space: That area perceived by the subject as being the space usually maintained between himself and another individual, and having its periphery identifed by means of a topographic device.

Perceived body space: That area perceived by the subject as being occupied by his body, and having its periphery identified by means of a topographic device.

Actual body space: That area occupied by the subject as determined by measurement of shoulder girdle width.

Hypotheses:

1. The higher the anxiety, the greater the difference between actual body space and perceived body space.
2. The higher the anxiety, the greater the difference between actual body space and perceived personal space.

3. The higher the anxiety, the greater the difference between perceived body space and perceived personal space.

INDEX

Action research
　aim of, 72
　contributions of, 72–73
　definition of, 72
　process of, 71–72
　rationale for, 71
Anxiety, Schlachter study of. *See* Schlachter (anxiety/personal space) study.
Axiom, definition of, 13

Bahnson (pathologic rhythm) theory, 57
Bentov consciousness index, 64

Concept, definition of, 7–8
Conceptual framework. *See also* Conceptual model.
　definition of, 5–6
　health-oriented. *See* Health, conceptualization of.
　purpose of, 6
　theory development within, 20–21

Conceptual model(s)
  definition of, 5–6
  differences in, 15
  of Johnson. *See* Johnson model.
  of Rogers. *See* Rogers model.
  of Roy. *See* Roy model.
  uses of, 15
Consciousness
  age and, 64
  correlates of, 66–67. *See also* Movement; Time.
  dimensions of, 64–66
  evolution of, 65–66
    animal studies of, 66
  expansion of, health and, 58
  index of, 64
  time and, 64
Construct(s)
  definition of, 8
  differences in, 41

Factors, inventory of
    consolidation in, 53
    developmental stages in, 45
    initial, 44–45
      diagrams of, 44, 46
    intervening variables in, 47
      diagram of, 48

Health, conceptualization of
    basic assumptions in, 56–58
    consciousness and. *See* Consciousness.
    dialectics in, 56
    dynamic relationships in, 55–56
    framework for, phenomenal selectivity in, 59

INDEX

Health, conceptualization of—*Continued*
  interrelationships in, 60
  movement component in, 61–63
  multidisciplinary contributions to, 73
  self-integration and, 58
  space-time component in, 61
  synthesis in, 56
Helson adaptation model, 17
Holism. *See* Nursing theory, holistic approach to.
Hypothesis, formulation of. *See* Theory, synthesis of.

Illness, conceptualization of. *See* Health, conceptualization of.
Interrelationship, law of
  examples of, 9, 10
  propositions and, 9
Intuition, theory development and, 43–44
Inventory, factor. *See* Factors, inventory of.

Johnson model, 3–4
  approach in, 19–20
  assessment basis in, 84
  assumptions of, 80–82
  focus of, 80
  framework of, 20–21
  goals in, 19, 82
  health-illness phenomena in, 19–20
  man-environment interaction in, 16–17
  nursing rationale in, 17–18, 83

Literature review
  factor identification in. *See* Factors, inventory of.
  intuition and, 43–44
  propositions derived from, 23–24
    in Schlachter study, 26–29

Maslow, phenomenological approach of, 70
Movement
　as communication, 62–63
　conceptualization of, 61–62
　self-awareness and, 62
　time experience and, 63

Newman (time perception) studies. *See also* Time, conceptualization of.
　axioms developed in, 49
　　diagram of, 50
　　　revised, 52
　intervening variables in, 47, 48, 51
　inventory of factors in
　　initial, 46–47
　　revised, 48
　perceived duration in, 51, 53
　propositions developed in, 51
　rationale for, 45
　testable relationship in, 47–48
　testable theorem in, 49
Nightingale, Florence, on nursing knowledge, 2
Nursing science
　fluid nature of, 7
　progress of, 73
Nursing theory. *See also* Theory.
　conceptual framework for. *See* Conceptual framework.
　conceptual models in. *See* Conceptual model.
　conceptualizations of
　　focus in, 55
　　overview of, 3–4
　criteria for, 2, 53
　definition of, 74
　developmental stages of, 2–3

INDEX

Nursing theory—*Continued*
  health component in. *See* Health, conceptualization of.
  holistic approach to
    action research in. *See* Action research.
    intraindividual change and, 70–71
    phenomenological component of, 70
    rationale for, 69–70
  Johnson model in. *See* Johnson model.
  literature review and. *See* Literature review.
  multivariate approach to, limitations of, 70
  nature of, 1–2
  prescriptive level component of, 2. *See also* Action research.
  research validation in, 23–24
  Rogers model in. *See* Rogers model.
  Roy model in. *See* Roy model.
  traditional methodology in, limitations of, 69

Ornstein (perceived duration) theory, 51, 53

Personal space, studies of. *See* Rodgers (personal space) study; Schlachter (anxiety/personal space) study.
Prescriptive level theory, 2, 72
Proposition(s). *See also* Relationships.
  axiomatic, 13
  definition of, 9
  literature review and. *See* Literature review.
  research supporting, 23
    ambiguities in, 24
  theorems as, 13

Relationships. *See also* Interrelationship, law of; Proposition(s).
  asymmetrical, 9–10
  correlational test of, 12

Relationships—*Continued*
　curvilinear, 10–11
　direction of, 9–10
　　erroneous, 12
　　interpretation of, 11–12
　symmetrical, 9–10
Research. *See also* Action research; Literature review.
　validation in, 23–24
Rodgers (personal space) study
　literature review in, propositions derived from, 36–37
　　　diagram of, 37
　main theory in, 37
　　diagram of, 38
　Schlachter study compared with, 40–41
　testable relationships in, 39
Rogers model, 3–4
　approach in, 20
　assessment basis in, 84
　assumptions of, 80–82
　focus of, 80
　framework of, 21
　goals in, 19, 82
　health-illness phenomena in, 20, 83
　man-environment interaction in, 16–17
　nursing rationale in, 18, 83
Roy model, 3–4
　approach in, 19
　assessment basis in, 84
　assumptions of, 81–82
　focus of, 80
　framework of, 20–21
　goals in, 19, 82
　health-illness phenomena in, 19, 83
　man-environment interaction in, 16–17
　nursing rationale in, 18, 83

INDEX

Schlachter (anxiety/personal space) study
  auxiliary theory in, 34, 36
    diagram of, 35
  constructs in, 25, 30, 85
  derived relationships in, 32
    objections to, 36
  hypotheses in, 85–86
  interrelationships in, 30
  literature review in, 25, 30
    axioms derived from, 32
      diagram of, 33
    propositions derived from, 26–29
      diagram of, 31
  main theory in, 32, 34
    diagram of, 35
  Rodgers study compared with, 40–41
  testable theorems developed in, 30, 32
  theoretical framework of, 25
    elimination process in, 30
Space-time, complementarity of, 61
Susman-Evered (action research) method. *See* Action research.

Theorem, definition of, 13
Theory
  holistic approach to. *See* Nursing theory, holistic approach to.
  synthesis of
    axiom formulation in, 49
      adjustments in, 50–51
      diagram of, 50
        revised, 52
    intuition in, 43–44
    methods of, 43
Time, conceptualization of

Time, conceptualization of—*Continued*
   age relationship in, 64
   consciousness index in, 64
   movement relationship in, 63
   space relationship in, 61

Variable(s). *See also* Factors, inventory of.
   definition of, 8